The Slim and Sane Solution

A Revolutionary Approach to Sustainable Fat Loss That Actually Works

Dortha Robel

ABOUT THE AUTHOR.

Dortha Robel, a qualified personal trainer and nutrition coach with over 10 years of experience in the fitness business, is the author of "The Thin and Sane Solution." Dortha is enthusiastic about assisting individuals in achieving their health and fitness objectives via a sustainable and practical approach to nutrition and exercise.

In her early twenties, Dortha became interested in health and fitness after struggling with her own weight and body image concerns. He attempted numerous fad diets and intense workout routines but found them to be unsustainable and harmful to her physical and emotional health. This experience inspired him to seek a career in the fitness sector, where he could assist others avoid the same problems and achieve long-term success.

Dortha has worked with individuals of various ages and fitness levels throughout the years, from elite athletes to busy working parents. He thinks that with the correct mentality, support, and direction, anyone can accomplish their health and fitness objectives. Her philosophy is built on the principals of balance, flexibility, and sustainability, and he seeks to encourage her clients to adopt beneficial lifestyle changes that they will be able to maintain for the rest of their lives.

Dortha is a trained yoga instructor and mindfulness practitioner in addition to her job as a personal trainer and nutrition consultant. He believes in the healing potential of holistic wellness and combines mindfulness and self-care practices into her coaching sessions.

Through "The Slim and Sane Solution," Dortha intends to reach a larger audience and assist more individuals accomplish their health and fitness objectives in a sustainable and sane manner.

Table of Contents

Introduction

The Problem with Traditional Diets.

Conventional diets have long been a well-liked method of losing weight since they frequently entail calorie restriction and/or severe restrictions on particular food categories. These diets can even be detrimental to a person's physical and mental health because they are frequently ineffectual.

Traditional diets frequently cannot be maintained over the long term, which is one of their primary drawbacks. Even if someone can lose weight at first, they frequently find it difficult to keep it off in the long run. This is because rigorous dietary limits included in conventional diets can produce feelings of deprivation and increased desires. This may set off a cycle of regaining weight and binge eating.

A person's physical health may also be harmed by traditional diets. Nutritional deficits brought on by calorie restriction can harm general health. Severe diets that restrict particular food categories can also result in nutritional intake imbalances and potentially raise the chance of developing certain medical conditions, such as osteoporosis and heart disease.

The mental health of a person might also be harmed by conventional diets. The emphasis on weight loss may result in an obsession with food and one's appearance, which may result in disordered eating patterns and a negative perception of one's body. An individual's self-esteem and general quality of life may suffer as a result.

Furthermore, standard diets frequently overlook the nuanced causes of weight gain, including hormone imbalances, stress, and sleep deprivation. It might be challenging to attain long-lasting weight reduction outcomes if one only concentrates on calorie restriction and food consumption, as this ignores other variables that may affect weight loss.

The Slim and Sane Solution: Overview

The Slim and Sane Solution is a ground-breaking method for losing weight in a healthy way that stresses a comprehensive approach. It is predicated on the notion that conventional eating routines, which frequently include calorie restriction and dietary limitations, are not long-term sustainable and may even be detrimental to a person's physical and mental health.

The Slim and Sane Solution concentrates on a more balanced method of weight management that considers unique issues including stress, sleep deprivation, and hormone imbalances. It places a strong emphasis on nutritious foods, intermittent fasting, and mindful eating as essential elements of a healthy and long-lasting weight management strategy.

The body receives necessary nutrients from whole meals, which are minimally processed and devoid of chemicals and preservatives. Whole foods also aid in controlling hunger and energy levels. It has been demonstrated that intermittent fasting, which includes decreasing food consumption for brief intervals, offers a number of health advantages, including enhanced insulin sensitivity and higher fat burning. Eating slowly and without interruptions while paying attention to hunger and fullness cues might assist to encourage healthy eating habits and prevent overeating.

The Slim and Sane Solution stresses the value of exercise, stress reduction, and self-care in addition to these dietary tactics for long-term weight loss. Exercise not only aids in calorie burning but also in muscle growth and general health improvement. Deep breathing and other stress-reduction practices, including meditation, can assist to lower stress levels and stop overeating. Overall health and wellness may be enhanced by engaging in self-care activities like obtaining enough sleep and practicing self-compassion.

How This Book Will Help You

The goal of the book "The Slim and Sane Solution: A New Method to Lasting Fat Reduction That Really Works" is to assist readers in achieving sustainable weight loss while also enhancing their general health and wellbeing.

A balanced approach to nutrition, exercise, stress management, and self-care is stressed throughout the book, which gives a thorough strategy to weight reduction that considers individual aspects including stress, sleep deprivation, and hormone imbalances.

The book will aid readers in understanding the science of fat reduction, including how calories, insulin, and hormones work, via thorough explanations and useful advice. A balanced and sustainable approach to nutrition, including whole foods, intermittent fasting, and mindful eating, will also be discussed in the book.

As important elements of a healthy and long-lasting approach to weight loss, the book also contains exercise regimens and techniques for stress management and self-care. Scientific research supports the techniques offered in the book, which are created to assist readers in achieving lasting fat reduction without experiencing deprivation or stress.

Part I

The Science of Sustainable Fat Loss

Chapter 1

Understanding the Basics of Fat Loss

Knowing the fundamentals of fat loss is critical for obtaining and maintaining a healthy weight. Fat loss happens when the body burns more calories than it intakes. This generates a calorie deficit, forcing the body to utilize stored fat for energy, resulting in weight reduction.

Diet, exercise, and metabolism are all important aspects in fat reduction. Consuming a well-balanced, low-calorie, high-nutrient diet is critical for fat loss. Eating less calories than the body requires can assist produce a calorie deficit, which can contribute to fat reduction.

Exercise is also beneficial for fat loss since it burns calories and increases metabolism. Frequent physical exercise can assist maintain muscular mass, which is vital for burning calories even when the body is at rest.

In addition to food and exercise, metabolism plays an important part in fat reduction. Metabolism refers to the body's capacity to transform food into energy.

A faster metabolism implies that the body consumes more calories even when at rest.

It is crucial to understand that fat loss is not the same as weight loss. Weight loss might include water weight, muscle loss, and fat loss. To accomplish long-term fat reduction, it is critical to focus on decreasing fat while maintaining muscle mass and general health.

What is Fat?

Adipose tissue, generally known as fat, is a complex and necessary component of the human body. It is a type of connective tissue that stores energy as triglycerides, which the body may break down and utilize as fuel.

In the body, there are two forms of fat: white fat and brown fat. The most prevalent form of fat is white fat, which is distributed throughout the body. Its principal role is to store energy and to keep the body warm. Brown fat, on the other hand, is present in modest deposits in the neck and upper back and serves primarily as a heat generator by burning calories.

Apart from energy storage, fat serves a variety of other functions in the body. Because some hormones are generated in fat cells, it is important in hormone control. Fat also cushions and protects important organs and aids in the regulation of body temperature.

While fat is an essential component of the human body, excess fat can cause a variety of health issues. Excess fat, especially visceral fat (fat surrounding the organs), has been related to an increased risk of heart disease, diabetes, and other chronic health problems.

Why Do We Gain Fat?

Genetics, nutrition, activity, and lifestyle are just a few of the many variables that might have an impact on how much weight you gain. Typically, when the body consumes more calories than it expends, fat is gained. A rise in total body fat results from the extra calories being deposited in fat cells.

Diet is a significant contributor to fat growth. Weight gain and a rise in body fat can result from consuming a diet high in calories, especially from meals that are high in fat and sugar. Extra fat can also be stored when a person consumes more calories than their body requires.

Lack of exercise is another important component in fat accumulation. The body burns less calories when it is not active, and extra calories may be turned into fat. A sedentary lifestyle can also result in muscle mass loss, which can further slow the metabolism and promote fat storage.

Moreover, genetics contribute to fat growth. Due to their genetic make-up, some people may be susceptible to gaining weight and storing fat more quickly than others. Yet, food and lifestyle choices may still have a big impact on an individual's weight and body fat %, therefore genetics may not always dictate these things.

Hormonal abnormalities can also play a role in fat gain. Insulin resistance, a condition in which the body becomes less sensitive to the hormone insulin, might, for example, contribute to increased fat accumulation. Other hormone abnormalities, such as cortisol, estrogen, and testosterone, can also lead to fat growth.

How Do We Lose Fat?

As the body burns more calories than it consumes, it loses fat, resulting in a drop in overall body fat. A multitude of factors, including nutrition, activity, and lifestyle, can all have an impact on the fat-loss process.

Creating a calorie deficit is an important aspect in fat loss. This can be accomplished by eating fewer calories than the body requires, increasing physical activity to burn more calories, or combining the two. For healthy and long-term fat loss, a moderate calorie deficit of 500-750 calories per day is usually suggested.

The content of the food is vital for fat reduction in addition to producing a calorie deficit. A high-protein, high-fiber diet can assist enhance satiety and promote fat reduction. Similarly, cutting less on processed meals, sugary beverages, and alcohol can help you lose weight.

Exercise is another crucial aspect of fat loss. Regular physical exercise can help the body burn more calories, resulting in more fat reduction. Strength training can also aid in the development of lean muscle mass, which can boost metabolism and aid in fat reduction.

In addition to food and exercise, stress management and good sleep are significant variables in fat reduction. Stress can cause the body to produce cortisol, a hormone that contributes to fat accumulation, whereas lack of sleep can disturb hormone balance and cause an increase in hunger and cravings.

Chapter 2

The Role of Nutrition in Fat Loss

Nutrition is important in fat reduction because it provides the body with the resources it needs to operate correctly and to boost fat burning activities. The most crucial component in fat reduction is creating a calorie deficit, which involves ingesting less calories than your body burns. To assist fat reduction and preserve general health, it is also necessary to ingest the proper sorts of nutrients in the right proportions.

Protein is an important macronutrient for fat reduction since it helps to sustain lean muscle mass and enhance metabolism. Protein-rich meals such as lean meats, fish, eggs, and plant-based sources such as beans and nuts will help you feel full and satisfied, as well as curb cravings for harmful foods.

Carbohydrates are also an essential macronutrient since they offer energy to the body for physical activity and exercise. Nevertheless, not all carbs are made equal, and it is critical to select complex carbohydrates that are high in fiber and slow to digest, such as whole grains, fruits, and vegetables.

Fats are frequently vilified when it comes to weight loss, although they are an essential component of a balanced diet. Good fats, such as those found in nuts, seeds, and avocados, can assist to improve hormone function and enhance feelings of fullness, which can help to lower overall calorie consumption.

In addition to macronutrients, micronutrients such as vitamins, minerals, and antioxidants are crucial for general health and can help with fat reduction by lowering inflammation and improving immunological function. Eating a variety of fruits and vegetables can assist to guarantee that you are getting a diverse range of micronutrients.

The Importance of Macronutrients

The body needs macronutrients in relatively significant amounts in order to operate effectively. They include lipids, proteins, and carbs, all of which are crucial for preserving general health and wellbeing.

The body's primary fuel source is carbohydrate. The body uses glucose, which is produced during their breakdown, as fuel. Many foods, such as fruits, vegetables, grains, and legumes, contain carbohydrates. It's crucial to take a healthy amount of carbs since an excess might result in weight gain and a deficiency can cause weariness.

Building and mending human tissues, particularly muscle tissue, depend on proteins. In addition, they are necessary for the creation of hormones, enzymes, and immune cells. Meat, fish, poultry, eggs, dairy products, beans, and legumes are all sources of protein. Protein has to be consumed in moderation since too much protein can harm the kidneys and too little protein can cause muscle loss.

The construction of cell membranes, the storage of energy, and the generation of hormones all depend on fats. They may also help some vitamins and minerals absorb better. Among the sources of good fats include nuts, seeds, avocados, olive oil, and oily salmon. Consuming the right quantity of fats is crucial since an imbalanced diet can result in vitamin deficits and weight gain and heart disease.

The Power of Micro-nutrients

Micronutrients are necessary nutrients that the body needs in minute quantities to operate properly. They all play significant roles in preserving general health and wellness, and they include vitamins, minerals, and trace elements.

Organic substances known as vitamins are not produced by the body and must be received from food. They are crucial for immune system health, energy generation, and general wellbeing. Fruits, vegetables, whole grains, and fortified foods are sources of vitamins.

The body requires trace amounts of minerals for healthy operation. Minerals are inorganic substances. They are crucial for maintaining the health of bones, nerves, and the body as a whole. Dairy goods, meats, fruits, and vegetables are all sources of minerals.

Although though trace elements are needed at much lower concentrations than other minerals, they are nevertheless necessary for optimal operation. Iron, zinc, and iodine are a few examples. These micronutrients are crucial for immunological health, the creation of energy, and general wellness.

To ensure optimal consumption of micronutrients, it's crucial to eat a balanced diet full of complete, nutrient-dense foods. To maintain optimal micronutrient consumption, several groups, including pregnant women, children, and the elderly, may necessitate extra supplements.

Anemia, a weaker immune system, and bone loss are just a few of the health complications that can result from micronutrient deficiencies. As a result, it's crucial to have a balanced diet and, if required, supplement with micronutrients while following the instructions of a healthcare professional.

How to Design a Sustainable Nutrition Plan

A long-term, fun, and useful strategy to healthy eating must be developed while designing a sustainable nutrition plan. While creating a sustainable nutrition plan, keep the following points in mind:

1. Identify your objectives: Establishing your goals is the first step in creating a nutrition

plan that is sustainable. Are you attempting to manage a medical condition, get healthier overall, gain muscle, or reduce weight? Setting objectives will enable you to customize your nutrition plan to meet your individual requirements.

2. Examine your present diet: It's crucial to evaluate your current eating patterns before making any dietary modifications. This is keeping track of the food you consume, figuring out if you're getting enough or too much of a certain nutrient, and documenting any bad eating habits.

3. Choose nutrient-dense foods: A sustainable nutrition strategy should be centered on nutrient-dense foods that offer a variety of macronutrients, vitamins, and minerals. They consist of lean protein sources, fruits, vegetables, whole grains, and healthy fats.

4. Avoid restrictive diets: Diets that significantly restrict calorie intake or remove whole food categories are not long-term maintainable. Instead, concentrate on eating in moderation and striking a healthy balance.

5. Prepare your meals: Making healthy food selections and time and money savings are two benefits of planning your meals ahead of time. To make eating healthy easier, think about prepping meals ahead of time or employing a meal delivery service.

6. Change your diet gradually: Changing your eating habits gradually is more sustainable than trying to completely change them all at once. Start by making minor adjustments, such as increasing the amount of fruits and vegetables in your meals or substituting water for sugary beverages.

7. Get expert advice: If you have certain dietary requirements or health issues, think about getting advice from a certified dietitian who can assist you in creating a sustainable nutrition plan that suits your unique requirements.

Chapter 3

The Role of Exercise in Fat Loss

Fat loss is greatly aided by exercise. By burning calories during exercise, you can establish a calorie deficit and lose weight. Yet exercising for fat loss has advantages that go beyond only burning calories.

The ability to build muscle mass is one of exercise's most important advantages. Due to its metabolic activity, muscle tissue burns calories even when you are not exercising. As a result, your body will burn more calories when at rest if you have higher muscle mass.

Building muscle mass can be significantly aided by strength training activities like weightlifting and bodyweight workouts. Running, cycling, and swimming are examples of cardiovascular workouts that can aid with fat burning and heart health.

Exercise also has the advantage of enhancing insulin sensitivity, which is crucial for controlling blood sugar levels. This indicates that your body is more adept at converting the carbs you ingest into energy rather than fat.

Moreover, physical activity can enhance general health and wellbeing. Frequent exercise has been associated with a lower chance of developing chronic conditions including diabetes, heart disease, and some forms of cancer. Also, it might lessen tension and lift one's spirits.

Exercise has the potential to be an immensely potent technique for attaining long-term fat loss when paired with a healthy, balanced diet. Finding an activity that you like and can fit into your lifestyle is crucial if you want to continue with it.

The Benefits of Exercise for Fat Loss

Each weight reduction regimen should include exercise since it increases calorie burn, builds lean muscle mass, and enhances general health. The following are some particular advantages of exercise for fat loss:

1. Improved calorie expenditure: Activity helps your body burn more calories throughout the day, which can help you achieve a calorie deficit and encourage fat reduction. Exercises that require a high level of intensity, like

weightlifting or interval training, can help you burn more calories.

2. Developing lean muscle mass: Weightlifting and other strength training activities can aid in the development of lean muscle mass, which can boost metabolism and encourage fat reduction. Having more muscle can help you burn more calories overall since muscular tissue burns more calories than fat tissue does.

3. Exercise can aid in improving insulin sensitivity, which is crucial for preserving stable blood sugar levels and encouraging fat reduction. Enhancing insulin sensitivity can also lower the danger of type 2 diabetes.

4. Decreased inflammation: It has been demonstrated that regular exercise helps to lower inflammation in the body, which is essential for general health and may help people lose weight.

5. Increased cardiovascular health: By fortifying the heart and enhancing circulation, exercise can enhance cardiovascular health. Also, it

can improve endurance and make it simpler to carry out everyday tasks.

6. Exercise has been demonstrated to lower stress levels, which can lower the risk of emotional eating and encourage the consumption of nutritious foods.

7. Exercise has been demonstrated to elevate mood and lessen anxiety and depressive symptoms. This might encourage commitment to and motivation in a weight loss program.

How to Design a Sustainable Exercise Plan

A sustainable fitness program must be created if you want to lose weight over the long run. Here are some important elements to take into account while creating a sustainable fitness program:

1. Set your goals first: Choose workouts that will assist you in achieving your unique weight reduction and fitness objectives. Think about your present level of fitness and any medical issues that could limit your capacity to exercise.

2. Choose activities you like: Choose workouts that suit your lifestyle and that you love doing. Long-term adherence to your fitness program will be simpler as a result.

3. Include different types of exercise: Include different types of exercise in your regimen, such as aerobic, weight training, and flexibility drills. This will keep you from becoming bored and guarantee that you are working out in all different ways.

4. Gradually up your intensity: As your fitness level increases, gradually lengthen and up your exercises' intensity. In addition to ensuring that you keep making progress, this will assist prevent injuries.

5. Plan your exercise routine: Make fitness a regular part of your schedule by scheduling your exercises at times that work for you. This will make it more likely that you'll follow through on your long-term fitness strategy.

6. Observe your body: Pay attention to how your body feels while exercising and after, and make any necessary adjustments to your strategy. This can entail changing your

workouts if you encounter pain or discomfort throughout your workouts or having a break day when you feel very exhausted.

7. Seek support: To help you stay motivated and accountable, think about hiring a personal trainer or enrolling in a fitness class.

The Importance of Recovery

Any lasting exercise regimen must include recovery as a key component. The methods and duration employed to provide the body the chance to recover from exercise are referred to. Recuperation is crucial for the following reasons:

1. Injury prevention: Recovery time is crucial to avoid injury since it enables the body to strengthen muscles and heal damaged tissues. Injury, tiredness, and burnout can result from overtraining without enough recuperation.

2. Enhances performance: Recovery time is crucial for enhancing athletic performance. The body may strengthen, become more flexible, and increase its resilience when

given enough time to heal. Improvements in stamina, quickness, and strength can result from this.

3. Reduces stress: Recovery can assist to minimize the stress that exercise can have on the body. Stretching, yoga, and meditation are among methods that can aid in promoting relaxation and lowering stress levels.

4. Improves overall health: Good recuperation can also improve one's health and wellbeing in general. It can strengthen the immune system, increase sleep quality, and lessen bodily inflammation.

5. Supports sustainability: Recovery is a crucial part of a fitness plan's sustainability. It is possible to avoid burnout and make it simpler to maintain a long-term exercise regimen by giving the body time to rest and recover.

Part II

The Slim and Sane Solution in Practice

Chapter 4

There are numerous crucial stages to starting the Slim and Sane Solution. Assessing your existing circumstances, including your eating habits, workout routine, and mentality, is the first step. This will assist you in determining your strengths and shortcomings as well as the areas where improvements need to be made.

Setting attainable, realistic goals is the next stage. These objectives must to be precise, quantifiable, and time-limited. Moreover, think about why you want to lose weight and concentrate on developing a strategy that will keep you dedicated and inspired throughout the procedure.

Creating a sustainable dietary plan is the next step after deciding on your goals. This strategy should be founded on the fundamentals of healthy eating, which include consuming nutrient-dense meals, getting enough protein, and balancing your intake of healthy fats and carbs. Also, things like meal preparation, time, and portion management should be taken into account.

The Slim and Sane Solution also emphasizes the need of exercise in addition to nutrition. Create a demanding yet realistic workout program that includes a range of exercises and activities to keep you interested and motivated. Your present level of fitness, any ailments or limits you may have, and your personal preferences should all be taken into account in the plan.

Lastly, healing, mentality, and balance should be emphasized. This entails including rest and recuperation days into your workout schedule, cultivating a good outlook and refraining from critical self-talk, and scheduling leisure time.

The Importance of Mindset

The ability to lose weight successfully and sustainably depends on one's mindset. It alludes to the thoughts and convictions that influence our behaviors and routines. Following are some main justifications for why mentality is significant:

1. Motivation: Adopting a positive outlook helps boost drive and dedication to weight reduction objectives. It may be simpler to maintain motivation and get beyond challenges if you concentrate on the advantages of healthy behaviors and a happy mindset.

2. Self-efficacy: The belief in one's capacity to accomplish goals may be strengthened by a sound attitude. In the face of difficulties, this can support the development of confidence and resilience.

3. Self-awareness: Self-awareness, or the capacity to comprehend one's own ideas, feelings, and behaviors, may also be influenced by mindset. We may make more deliberate judgments and form healthier habits by being aware of the elements that affect our habits and choices.

4. Persistence is essential for overcoming obstacles and attaining long-term success. A growth mindset can help people be more persistent and resilient. It might be simpler to maintain commitment to weight reduction

objectives over time if you concentrate on progress rather than perfection.

5. Stress reduction: Having a positive outlook can also help you feel less stressed, which might hinder your attempts to lose weight. Stress management and maintaining focus on good behaviors may be made simpler by engaging in mindfulness and positive thinking exercises.

How to Set Realistic Goals

To lose weight successfully and sustainably, reasonable goals must be set. The following are important actions for developing realistic goals:

1. Be explicit: Well stated, detailed goals are best. Try creating a precise goal, such as "drop 10 pounds in 3 months," rather than a general one like "lose weight."

2. Be reasonable: Objectives must to be doable and reasonable. Establishing an impossible or unreasonable objective can cause disappointment and frustration.

3. Be quantifiable: In order to measure progress, goals should be measurable. Setting particular goals, such as weight loss, measurement reduction, or body fat percentage, can help with this.

4. Be time-bound: Objectives have to have a deadline for fulfillment. This may increase motivation and a sense of urgency about completing the task.

5. Set smaller, more manageable goals: Larger objectives can be more easily attained and assist to create momentum if they are divided into smaller, more manageable tasks.

6. Celebrating accomplishments may help you stay motivated and boost your confidence. Setting up modest prizes for attaining along the way milestones is one method to do this.

7. Be flexible: Objectives should be adaptive to alterations in the environment. This can lessen frustration and make room for any necessary modifications.

To have long-lasting effects, it's crucial to set up your environment for weight reduction success. To get your surroundings ready, consider these suggestions:

1. Get rid of harmful snacks and items that can be tempting to indulge in to remove temptation. Stock your kitchen instead with wholesome, nutrient-dense meals that help you achieve your weight loss objectives.

2. Plan your meals: Making a mental note of what you're going to eat will help you avoid impulsive, unhealthy decisions and make sure that you have healthy options available.

3. Maintain a supply of nutritious snacks: Have wholesome snacks like fruits, veggies, and nuts close at hand. By doing so, you can avoid munching unhealthily and stave off hunger.

4. Make exercise accessible: Look for methods to make exercise simple and available. This might entail establishing a home gym,

locating a workout partner, or enrolling in a fitness class or gym in the neighborhood.

5. Establish a positive atmosphere by surrounding yourself with friends and family who will assist you in achieving your weight reduction objectives.

6. Follow your development: Use a food diary or weight loss app to monitor your progress. This might serve to hold you accountable and inspire you to continue succeeding.

7. Self-awareness and mindfulness exercises might help you better understand your triggers and patterns. This can assist you in seeing possible obstacles and proactively altering your surroundings to support your objectives.

Chapter 5

The Slim and Sane Solution Meal Plan is a step-by-step approach to eating a healthy, balanced diet for long-term fat loss. The meal plan is based on the macronutrient balance, portion management, and inclusion of a variety of complete, nutrient-dense foods principles.

The meal plan is intended to be adjustable to individual tastes and dietary limitations. It contains a wide variety of foods, such as lean proteins, healthy fats, complex carbohydrates, fruits, and vegetables.

The daily food plan includes three main meals (breakfast, lunch, and supper) as well as two snacks. Each meal and snack is designed to offer a macronutrient balance (protein, carbs, and fats) to promote energy levels, muscle repair, and fat reduction.

To assist readers keep on track with their dietary objectives, the meal plan also provides meal preparation and portion management advice. It highlights the significance of meal planning and preparation ahead of time in order to avoid bad food choices and foster healthy behaviors.

A healthy and sustainable meal plan is centered on supplying the body with the nutrition it need while also supporting weight loss objectives. Here are a few crucial guidelines for creating a great food plan:

1. Incorporate a range of nutrient-dense foods in your diet: Include a variety of full, nutrient-dense foods including fruits, vegetables, lean meats, healthy fats, and whole grains in your diet.

2. Limit portion sizes: While including a variety of meals is vital, it's equally necessary to regulate portion sizes to support weight reduction objectives. To guarantee accurate portion amounts, use measuring cups and spoons or a food scale.

3. Balance macronutrients: To support general health and weight reduction objectives, balance macronutrients such as protein,

carbs, and fat. With each meal, strive for a balance of all three.

4. Add fiber-rich foods such as fruits, vegetables, and whole grains in your diet to promote satiety and digestive health.

5. Restrict or eliminate added sugars and highly processed meals, which can lead to weight gain and other health problems.

6. Make a plan: Prepare ahead of time for meals and snacks to ensure that healthy selections are easily available and to avoid impulsive, unhealthy choices.

7. Hydrate correctly: Hydration is essential for general health and weight reduction. Drink lots of water throughout the day and minimize your intake of sugary drinks and alcohol.

Sample Meal Plan

Lean protein, healthy fats, whole grains, and an abundance of fruits and vegetables might be included in an example meal plan for weight loss and overall health. A daily food plan sample is shown below:

Breakfast:

- Oatmeal with almond milk, topped with sliced banana, chia seeds, and a drizzle of honey
- 1 hard-boiled egg

Mid-morning snack:

- Apple slices with almond butter

Lunch:

- Grilled chicken breast with roasted vegetables (such as sweet potato, zucchini, and bell pepper)
- Quinoa or brown rice
- Mixed greens salad with vinaigrette dressing

Afternoon snack:

- Greek yogurt with mixed berries

Dinner:

- Baked salmon with lemon and herbs
- Roasted Brussels sprouts with garlic

- 1/2 cup of wild rice

Evening snack:

- Small bowl of mixed nuts

This meal plan provides a variety of nutrient-dense foods while controlling portion sizes and limiting added sugars and processed foods. It includes fiber-rich foods, such as fruits and vegetables, to promote satiety and digestive health. Additionally, this plan includes protein with every meal to support muscle growth and repair, healthy fats for satiety and brain health, and whole grains for sustained energy throughout the day.

Tips for Meal Planning and Preparation

Planning and preparing meals are essential steps in achieving weight reduction goals and leading a healthy lifestyle. Here are some ideas to aid you with meal planning and preparation:

1. Plan ahead by setting some time each week to prepare your meals and snacks. You can keep organized and make sure you have

access to healthy food selections by doing this.

2. Meal preparation: Make a plan for the entire weeks' worth of meals. By eliminating last-minute excursions to the grocery store and fast food runs, you can save time and money by doing this.

3. Prepare a list of the ingredients you'll need for your meals and snacks and take it to the store. Keep to your list to prevent impulsive purchases.

4. To save time during dinner preparation, prepare items in advance. Cut vegetables, boil grains, and marinade meats.

5. Cook in bulk: Make a lot of casseroles, soups, and stews that you can divide out and freeze for later use.

6. Employ measuring cups or a food scale to measure out your meals and snacks to practice portion management. By doing this, you may prevent overeating and make sure that you are staying inside your calorie budget.

7. Preparing your meals and snacks in advance will help you have access to a variety of healthful foods when you're out and about.

8. Invest in dependable containers for storage if you want to keep your food accessible and fresh.

9. To keep your meals fresh and fulfilling, don't be scared to experiment. Test out different recipes and ingredients.

10. Maintain flexibility: Be adaptable with your food plan and ready to make changes as necessary. Plans may alter as a result of life.

Chapter 6

The Slim and Sane Solution Exercise Plan

To assist people in achieving their fat reduction objectives, the Slim and Sane Solution Workout Plan is a complete program that incorporates flexibility exercises, weight training, and aerobic exercise. The program is intended to assist people in achieving their ideal level of fitness while also being sustainable, entertaining, and successful.

Beginner, intermediate, and advanced phases make up the fitness program. As the person advances, the intensity and complexity of each phase steadily grow during its four-week duration.

By include bodyweight exercises, low-impact aerobic training, and basic stretches, the novice phase concentrates on building a strong foundation of fitness. This phase aims to increase strength and endurance while being accessible to people of all fitness levels.

By adding more difficult workouts, such weightlifting and greater intensity cardiovascular training, the intermediate phase strengthens the foundation created in the novice phase. This phase aims to improve a person's general fitness level, cardiovascular endurance, and muscular mass.

The most difficult section of the workout is the advanced phase, which is intended for people who have previously developed a solid base of fitness. To assist people continue to challenge themselves and reach their fat reduction objectives, this phase includes high-intensity interval training, advanced weightlifting methods, and more difficult stretches.

The training regimen stresses the value of recovery and rest at every stage. Rest days are incorporated into the schedule to give the body time to recuperate and avoid damage.

The Slim and Sane Solution Workout Plan offers advice on how to adjust the schedule to suit unique requirements and tastes. It also offers suggestions for adding outdoor activities and group fitness courses into the plan, as well as choices for adapting workouts for people with injuries or physical limitations.

The following guidelines should be kept in mind while creating an exercise program:

1. Exercise should be done often, ideally at least three to five times each week. The secret to getting results is consistency.

2. Workout should be done at a moderate to high intensity to push your body and encourage fitness progress. This can be done by putting on more weight or resistance, going faster, or using more intense intervals.

3. Time: For best outcomes, exercise sessions should last at least 30 minutes but better 45 to 60 minutes.

4. Type: Exercise should incorporate both aerobic and resistance training to improve flexibility, muscular strength, and all other components of fitness.

5. To prevent reaching a plateau and keep experiencing gains, exercise should be gradually increased in intensity, duration, and/or frequency.

6. Recovery: To avoid injury and to provide the body enough time to regenerate muscle tissue, rest and recovery time are crucial. This involves getting enough sleep and having rest days.

7. Enjoyment: Workout ought to be pleasurable and enduring. To guarantee that you remain with your workout regimen over time, find activities that you love and that fit into your lifestyle.

Sample Exercise Plan

Monday:

- Warm-up with five to ten minutes of gentle cardio (e.g. walking, jogging, cycling)
- 3 sets of 8–12 repetitions each of squats, lunges, chest presses, shoulder presses, and rows make up resistance training.
- 20 to 30 minutes of moderate-intensity exercise for cardiovascular training (e.g. cycling, rowing, elliptical)
- Stretching for 5 to 10 minutes as a cool-down

Tuesday:

- Rest day or low-intensity exercise (such as yoga or strolling)

Wednesday:

- Warm-up with five to ten minutes of gentle cardio
- 3 sets of 8–12 repetitions each of the following exercises: pushups, deadlifts, leg presses, bicep curls, and tricep extensions
- 20 to 30 minutes of high-intensity interval exercise for the heart (e.g. sprints, stair-climbing)
- Stretching for 5 to 10 minutes as a cool-down

Thursday:

- A day of rest or little exercise

Friday:

- Warm-up with five to ten minutes of gentle cardio
- Step-ups, calf raises, lat pull-downs, chest flies, and reverse fly's are included in three

sets of eight to twelve repetitions of resistance training.

- Training for the heart: 20 to 30 minutes of steady-state exercise (e.g. jogging, swimming, cycling)
- Stretching for 5 to 10 minutes as a cool-down

Saturday:

- Rest day or little exercise:

Sunday:

- Warm-up with five to ten minutes of gentle cardio
- Exercises for the core, lateral raises, upright rows, and hamstring curls, all performed in three sets of eight to twelve repetitions each (e.g. planks, crunches)
- cardio-vascular exercise 20 to 30 minutes of cardio at a moderate intensity
- Stretching for 5 to 10 minutes as a cool-down

While creating an exercise regimen, there are a few crucial considerations to keep in mind to ensure that it is effective, safe, and long-term. Here are some pointers to help you plan and carry out your workout routine:

1. Start slowly and gradually increase intensity: Whether you're new to exercising or returning after a break, it's critical to begin softly and gradually raise the intensity over time. This will help you prevent injury and keep you on track with your strategy.

2. Pick activities you enjoy: Exercise should be something you look forward to doing. This increases the likelihood that you will adhere to your strategy in the long run. Try out several hobbies to see what you like most, whether it's jogging, swimming, dancing, or weight lifting.

3. Change your routine: Performing the same workouts every day might get monotonous and may lead to a plateau in your results. Include a variety of workouts and activities

into your regimen, such as cardio, weight training, and flexibility work.

4. Make time for recovery: Recovery is a critical component of any fitness program. Include rest days and healing exercises like foam rolling or stretching.

5. Establish realistic goals: Create objectives for yourself that are reasonable and attainable, such as increasing the amount of weight you can lift or running a specific distance in a given period of time. This will keep you motivated and allow you to monitor improvement over time.

6. Track your progress: Keep tabs on your development by recording your exercises and performance. You may use this to praise your accomplishments and pinpoint areas that need improvement.

7. Work with a professional: To help you create and carry out an efficient strategy, consider working with a licensed personal trainer or exercise expert if you are new to exercising or have special goals. They may provide you

advice on good form, growth, and accountability.

Chapter 7

Staying Sane While Losing Fat

Fat loss may be a difficult and emotional struggle. It necessitates discipline, dedication, and consistency, all of which can be difficult to sustain. As a result, it's critical to focus your mental health and well-being throughout this process. Here are some suggestions for keeping sane while reducing weight:

Self-care: Make an effort to look after yourself both physically and psychologically. This might include getting adequate sleep, taking pauses when required, and engaging in enjoyable activities.

Concentrate on progress rather than perfection: Don't berate yourself if you have setbacks or slip-ups. Instead, concentrate on your accomplishments and use them as incentive to keep going.

Surround yourself with people who support you: Seek the help of friends, family, or a group that shares your aims. Having a support network can help you stay motivated and accountable.

Integrate mindfulness techniques, such as meditation or yoga, into your daily routine. These can assist you in remaining present and reducing tension and worry.

Appreciate non-scale victories: Avoid focusing entirely on the number on the scale. Some achievements to celebrate include increasing strength or endurance or fitting into a lower size of clothing.

Avoid making comparisons: Remember that everyone's experience is different, and comparing yourself to others may be detrimental. Concentrate on your own progress and ambitions.

The Importance of Balance and Flexibility

A well-rounded workout regimen must include both balance and flexibility. This is why:

1. Balance is essential for everyday actions such as walking, standing, and climbing stairs. It also becomes more essential as we become older since it can assist prevent falls and lower the chance of damage. Balance exercises can help you improve your balance and stability by including them into your training program.

2. Flexibility is essential for preserving mobility and avoiding injury. Muscle imbalances and compensations caused by a lack of flexibility might increase the risk of injury. Stretching and mobility exercises can help you increase your flexibility and decrease your risk of injury.

3. Posture Improvement: Excellent balance and flexibility can help you improve your posture. Bad posture can cause a variety of problems, such as back discomfort, neck pain, and headaches. You may assist maintain good alignment and lessen the likelihood of these disorders by increasing your balance and flexibility.

4. Stress Reduction: Balancing and flexibility activities like yoga and tai chi can also help decrease stress and enhance general well-being. Deep breathing, awareness, and relaxation are the emphasis of these exercises, which can help decrease stress and enhance mental health.

Integrating balance and flexibility exercises into your workout program does not have to be difficult. Standing on one leg, lunges, and stretching are all simple workouts that can help you improve your balance and flexibility. Try adding a yoga or tai chi lesson to your program for a more disciplined approach.

Strategies for Dealing with Setbacks

Setbacks are unavoidable in any weight reduction or fitness endeavor. These might be irritating, but keep in mind that setbacks do not define your development. These are some ways to deal with setbacks:

1. Self-Compassion: It is critical to be compassionate to oneself when you experience failures. Avoid negative self-talk and self-criticism. Instead, exercise self-compassion by treating oneself with the same care, concern, and understanding that you would show a good friend.

2. Setbacks may be used to learn and progress. Take some time to think about what occurred

and what you can do differently next time. Maybe you need to change your diet or exercise routine, or maybe you need to concentrate on developing new habits. Utilize the setback to discover areas for improvement.

3. Reframe Your Thinking: Instead of perceiving setbacks as failures, attempt to reframe them as chances for progress. Setbacks may be used to improve resilience and tenacity. Accept the challenge and utilize it as fuel to keep moving forward.

4. Seek Help: Having a support system may be quite beneficial while dealing with difficulties. Get the advice and assistance of a friend, family member, or professional. Participating in a support group or working with a coach or trainer may also help with accountability and motivation.

5. Establish Reasonable Goals: When ambitions are too ambitious or unrealistic, setbacks might arise. Spend some time re-evaluating your goals to ensure they are attainable and sustainable. Scale down

bigger ambitions into smaller, more doable actions.

6. Celebrate Progress: It is critical to recognize and celebrate progress, no matter how modest. Take some time to reflect on your success thus far and use it as motivation to keep going.

How to Stay Motivated and Focused

While attempting to attain a long-term objective such as consistent fat reduction, staying motivated and focused can be difficult. There are, however, several tactics that can help you stay on track and motivated throughout the process:

1. Establish explicit, quantifiable, and achievable objectives: Make your goals clear and measurable so you can measure your progress and celebrate your accomplishments. Setting a target of losing 1-2 pounds every week, for example, is concrete, measurable, and attainable.

2. Discover your "why": Knowing why you want to attain your objective will help you stay

motivated during difficult times. Ask yourself why you want to lose weight and remind yourself of your motivations on a frequent basis.

3. Little victories should be celebrated: Small victories along the road might help you keep motivated and focused on your long-term goals. For example, after reaching a specified weight reduction goal or finishing a difficult workout.

4. Surround yourself with people who will support you: Having a support system of family, friends, or a coach may help you stay accountable and motivated. Communicate your aims with them and solicit their assistance as required.

5. Continue to learn and evolve: Always studying about diet, exercise, and mentality may help you stay involved and motivated. Try with new healthy foods, fitness routines, and inspiring podcasts or audiobooks.

6. Take care of your physical and mental health: Taking care of your physical and mental health is vital for keeping motivated and

focused. Prioritize getting adequate sleep, reducing stress, and engaging in self-care activities that you like.

Conclusion

Recap of the Slim and Sane Solution

The Slim and Sane Solution is an all-encompassing plan for long-term fat loss that places a strong emphasis on healthy eating, consistent activity, and a good outlook. Without turning to fad diets or drastic methods, the approach is intended to assist people in losing weight in a healthy and long-lasting way.

A variety of subjects are covered in the book, such as the science of fat reduction, the significance of macro- and micronutrients, the advantages of exercise and recuperation, and the relevance of mentality in attaining success. It offers helpful advice on how to make a long-term dietary plan, build a schedule of exercise that is unique to you, and set up your surroundings for success.

The necessity of making sensible objectives, coping with failures, and maintaining motivation and focus are also emphasized in the book. Together with recommendations for food planning and preparation, exercise planning and execution, and preserving balance and flexibility, it offers sample meal plans and exercise regimens.

How to Maintain Your Results

It might be as crucial to maintain your results after accomplishing your fat reduction objectives as it can be to actually accomplish those objectives. It necessitates a dedication to upholding healthy routines and adopting long-lasting lifestyle modifications. Here are some pointers for keeping your outcomes:

1. After achieving your fat reduction objectives, it's crucial to keep up with a balanced diet that contains lots of fruits, vegetables, lean meats, and healthy fats. This will promote general health and assist in maintaining a healthy weight.

2. Maintain a regular exercise schedule: Maintaining a healthy weight, developing strength and endurance, and sustaining general health all depend on frequent exercise. Strive to keep up the workout regimen that helped you reach your fat

reduction objectives or look for new things to do to stay motivated.

3. Create new objectives: Refining your exercise or health goals will help you stay motivated and focused on advancing. This can entail preparing for a fresh fitness challenge, trying a brand-new sport or activity, or concentrating on increasing strength or endurance.

4. Self-care: Taking care of your mental and emotional wellness is essential for long-term success. To assist manage stress and support general well-being, engage in self-care activities such as meditation, yoga, or other relaxation techniques.

5. Seek out a supporting community of friends, family, or a fitness club to help you keep motivated and accountable. Consider hiring a personal trainer or nutritionist to assist you in maintaining your success and making healthy decisions.